GAPS DIET

Recipes for Rapid

Gut Repair

(**Stages 1-6**)

purview. There are no scenarios in which the publisher or the original author of this work can be in any fashion deemed liable for any hardship or damages that may befall them after undertaking information described herein.

Additionally, the information in the following pages is intended only for informational purposes and should thus be thought of as universal. As befitting its nature, it is presented without assurance regarding its prolonged validity or interim quality. Trademarks that are mentioned are done without written consent and can in no way be considered an endorsement from the trademark holder.

TABLE OF CONTENTS

Introduction

Over 2,000 years ago Hippocrates proclaimed that "all disease beings in the gut", and according to Huffington Post, "it's common to overlook the health of our gastrointestinal system, even though it contains 10-times more health-determining bacteria than the rest of our body." Most people have a healthy balance of bacteria in their system, but a lack of bacterial diversity. Western society treats any malady with medications, and as a collective we take a lot of pills for a lot of problems: medications like antibiotics, birth control, anti-depressants, antacids, etc. Chronic stress and exposure to environmental toxins can also alter digestive secretions, gut permeability, blood flow, and diet sensitivity.

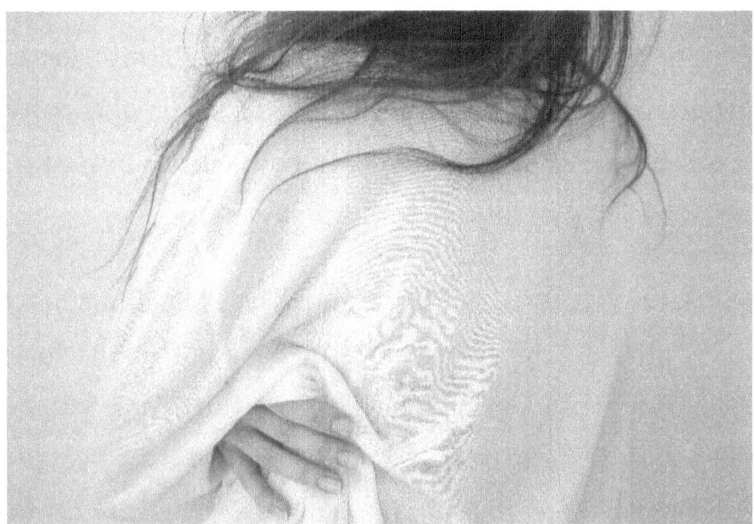

Photo by Daria Nepriakhina on Unsplash

While our stomachs are considered an external organ, they are housed inside our bodies and their job is to protect us from harmful substances that try to enter our bodies. Trillions of bacteria can be found inside our bodies, and that bacteria play an important role in how well or poor our bodies function. When this bacterium gets paired with other viruses and fungi in your system, they become known as microbiota, and each person's makes up a unique environment. Our intestines and colon are lined with millions of bacteria that play a role in our metabolic function and hardiness of our immune system. While we have a lot of bacteria all throughout the body, it is specifically the bacteria in our digestive systems that can have a direct link to our health and well being.

People who experience illnesses and diseases often have an imbalance of bacteria: sometimes there is too much of one type, or they are lacking a diversity of bacteria to begin with. Research has been conducted that has been able to connect dots between diseases, illnesses, and the bacteria content of your gut; that bacteria can have an impact on the following:

- Heart disease, diabetes, and obesity. Metabolic function is affected by the bacteria in your gut in the form of calories used from food and the nutrient content the body receives from said food. Bacteria in excess can cause fiber in your gut to turn into fatty acids, leading to fat deposit build-up in your liver, which can lead to metabolic syndrome.

- Inflammatory diseases of the bowl such as Crohn's disease and ulcerative colitis. It's hypothesized that people who suffer from these kinds of ailments are missing key anti-inflammatory gut bacteria that may cause the body to begin attacking your own intestines.
- Autism, anxiety, and depression. Nerve endings in the gut communicate with your brain, also known as the gut-brain-axis. Studies have suggested that a link exists between gut health and central nervous system disorders.
- Arthritis
- Colon cancer

The GAPS Diet can assist in the healing of your gut which may lead to the remission or disappearance of symptoms. The diet hypothesizes that when you focus on improving gut health, leaky gut syndrome which can lead to many of the above ailments, can be cured by fortifying your gut microbiota to decrease permeability and the leaking of toxins into the bloodstream. This is a healing protocol that can fix gut ailments, reduce inflammation, and potentially treat certain conditions that have manifested in the brain, but that begin in the stomach.

The diet puts an emphasis on foods that are good for the gut and high in nutrients, and the elimination of several food groups that are hard on the digestive system. Limited research exists out there about the GAPS Diet and whether or not it can back up its touted benefits, but either way it is clear that bacterial health in the gut can play a large role in many aspects of a person's health. There are, however, many studies that can back the individual components of the GAPS Diet and those studies show that following one or more of the components of the diet can lead to a slew of health benefits.

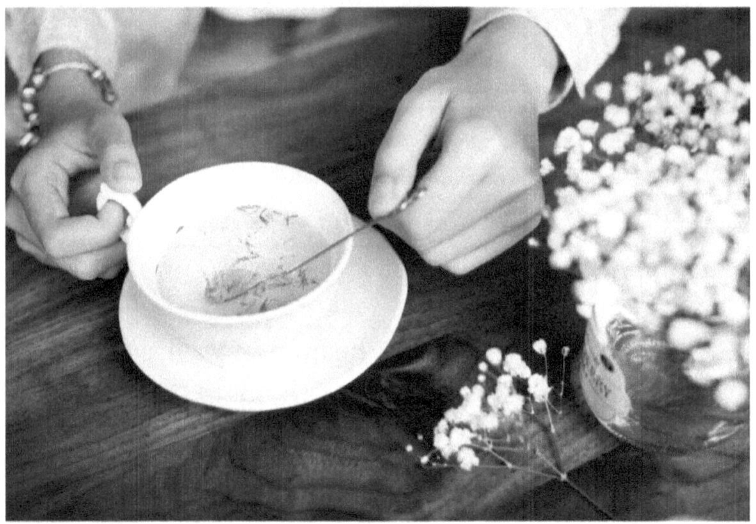

Photo by rawpixel on Unsplash

It is recommended that you implement the introduction portion of the diet first, before jumping into the Full GAPS Diet, but if you do not suffer from severe digestive issues or food sensitivities, you can, probably, very easily jump straight into the Full Diet. Supplementation is also an important part of the diet, and mainly include the use of a high-quality probiotic. Make sure you research different brands before purchasing, many do not deliver the strength or bacteria variety that the bottle claims to deliver. To find a good probiotic make sure you look for the following characteristics:

- A variety of beneficial bacteria species
- Different groups of probiotic bacteria in several strains
- A concentrated number of bacteria, preferably close to 8 million bacteria
- Tested by the manufacturer for strength and bacterial composition in each batch with published results

Other important supplements on the diet include vitamin and mineral supplements, Vitamin A, essential fatty acids, AND digestive enzymes as needed for your individual body and digestive health needs. Detoxifying can be difficult and can cause damage to the body on top of its accumulated toxins. Supporting the body's natural detoxification process helps repair damaged tissues.

Many people are dissatisfied with more traditional and available treatments for disorders like autism and are looking for new ways to attempt to treat their disease and symptoms. Those who give the diet a chance normally see a cessation of food intolerances and sensitivities, and sometimes even a full recovery from their ailment. You will find people out there who have tried the diet and claim that it does not work, and in fact, it may not have worked for them, but for better or for worse you will most likely come out at the other end of the diet feeling slightly better if not completely better just from eliminating many sources of food that are not optimal for our systems in general like highly-processed, sugar-laden fast foods, and packaged foods.

There is no guarantee that trying out the GAPS Diet will cure your ailments, and while there is no guarantee, there is no harm in trying out the diet in order to heal your gut. Approaching this diet with an open mind could potentially lead to dramatic health improvements like the total removal of allergies or skin conditions. This diet may not be suitable for everyone, such as vegetarians or vegans who may struggle to meet their nutritional needs based on the approved foods list because the diet relies heavily on products derived from animals.

The GAPS Diet should not replace your current medication or treatments of conditions, but should be used in conjunction with traditional treatments to improve your gut health. Always consult the advice of a certified health care professional if you suffer from a pre-existing condition before you start the GAPS Diet. If your doctor does not recommend that you adhere to the GAPS Diet, you can always do it in a modified form like excluding carbs, or sugars, or grains instead of all of them at the same time and see what happens to your digestive system.

CHAPTER 1: WHAT IS THE GAPS DIET?

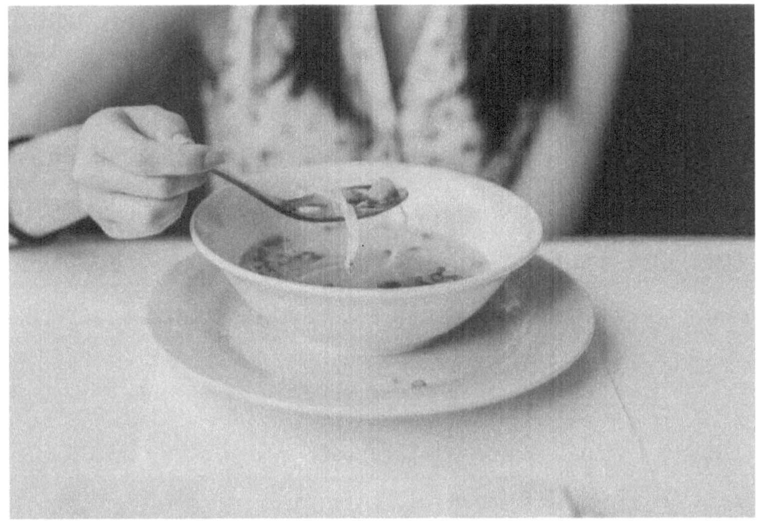

Photo by Henrique Félix on Unsplash

What is the GAPS Diet? GAPS Diet, was originally based off of the Specific Carbohydrate Diet (SCD Diet) by Dr. Sidney Valentine Hass in the 1920s in an attempt to heal digestive disorders like inflammatory bowel disease and leaky gut syndrome. Today, the GAPS Diet claims to treat anything from autism, to ADHD, depression, and anxiety. This diet puts an emphasis on foods that are easy to digest and that are also very high in nutrients, and replacing our normal grains, starchy vegetables, and refined carbs from our typical diet with good-for-our-stomach foods.

The meal plan for the diet is broken down into six stages, with stage one being the most restrictive. As with many other diets, key foods are slowly added back in to your diet plan as you progress through stages. Gut health is an important aspect of health, but only limited research exists on the benefits and the outcomes of the GAPS Diet.

The creator of the GAPS Diet, Dr. Campbell-McBride has the theory that many gut health conditions are related to brain function, and brain function is related to gut health. One main cause of many issues is leaky gut syndrome which describes the increasing permeability of the gut wall.

The theory hypothesizes that a leaky gut allows chemicals and bacteria from your food and environment to enter into your blood steam, and when they do they can negatively affect your brain function and development leading to symptoms like brain fog. Our gastrointestinal tract plays a very important role in our overall health and functioning of digestion, nutrient absorption, immune system response, hormone regulation, detoxification, elimination, and the production of energy. The GAPS Diet is designed to heal this gut permeability and prevent toxins from entering the body.

Many people attempt to cut out unprocessed foods when they start to succumb to health issues, and a widely accepted step toward addressing those issues focuses on an elimination diet. While this can lead finding the culprit of your woes, it usually does not go that extra step to heal the body and reverse the damage that has been caused.

Along with leaky gut, nutrient deficiencies and imbalanced gut flora (gastrointestinal microbiota) imbalances can also be addressed by following the GAPS Diet. The diet eliminates the consumption of bad-for-you foods such as any foods that are canned, processed, sweet, or fast foods, and encourages an organic diet rich in vegetables, fish, etc. with the goal of introducing good bacteria to the body to help cleanse out the toxins.

The diet can be a year-long process, and is most often used for children, although it can absolutely be modified for short-term usage and adults. The GAPS protocol is broken down into three main stages:

1. Introduction phase
2. Full GAPS diet phase
3. Reintroduction phase

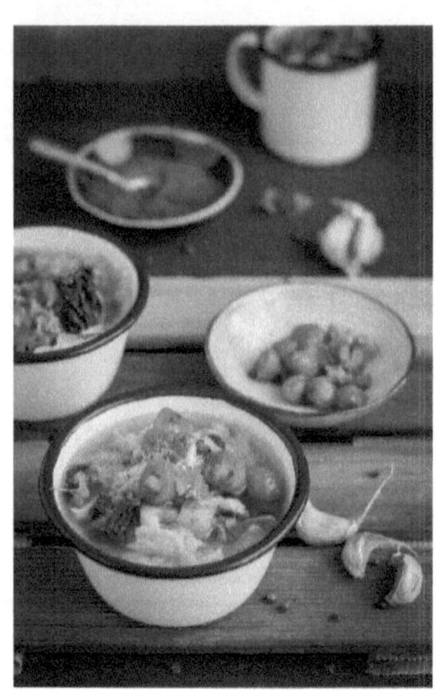

The Introduction phase revolves around the concept of elimination: during this phase you eliminate foods like starchy carbs, and instead you will eat mostly broths, stews, and probiotic foods before you slowly start to add in foods in the following stages:

- Stage 1: consuming homemade bone broth, juice from probiotic foods and ginger, and unpasteurized, homemade yogurt or kefir.

- Stage 2: add in raw organic egg yolks, ghee, and stews made with vegetables and meat or fish.

- Stage 3: all previous foods plus avocado, fermented vegetables, duck or goose fat.

- Stage 4: add in grilled and roasted meats, olive oil (preferably cold-pressed), vegetable juice, and bread prepared using an approved GAPS recipe.

- Stage 5: introduce cooked apple puree, raw vegetables starting with lettuce and peeled cucumber, fruit juice, and small amounts of citrus based raw fruits.
- Stage 6: introduce more raw fruit and citrus fruits

The full GAPS Diet phase can last anywhere from 1-3 years depending on the changes you want to see. The majority of a person's diet during this time will consist mostly on the following foods:

- Fresh meat, preferably hormone-free and grass-fed
- Animals fats
- Fish including shellfish
- Organic eggs
- Fermented foods
- Vegetables

The reintroduction phase starts the time when you can start reintroducing some of the prohibited foods back into your diet. This phase is recommended after you have been regularly experiencing normal digestion, and each food is gradually introduced individually and with increasing portions. Start small, by adding the food in 1-2 teaspoons at a time, work your way up to tablespoons, and then eventually to whole foods. Even when off the diet it is suggested that you not continue to eat any highly-processed and refined, high-sugar foods.

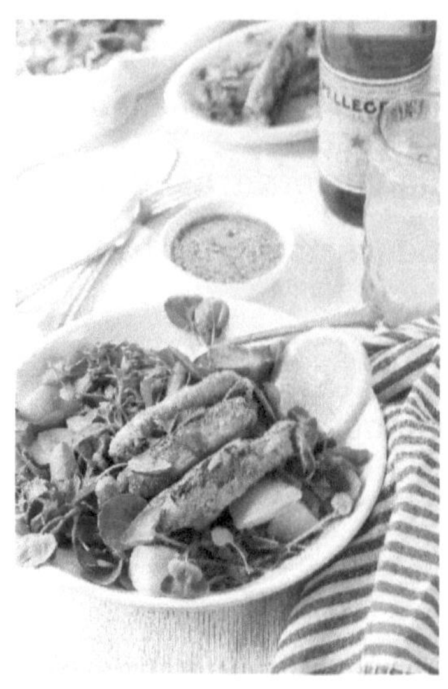

Photo by Lauren Lester on Unsplash

Purposefulnutrition.com interviewed several people who have tried their hand at the GAPS Diet over the years, and the following is an interview given by a woman named Debbie, a blogger at "The Sour Path is the Sweetest." It is about her experience with the diet and what led her to give it a try in the first place:

"Question: How long have you been on the GAPS diet?
Answer: Almost 3 years. I started in October 2010."

"Question: What was going on that made you decide to pursue the diet?
Answer: I had severe depression, anxiety, and a diagnosis of bipolar disorder with mixed states. For some reason, all medicines and most supplements made me feel worse because

I'm weirdly sensitive. I also was freezing! My body temp would drop to 94 degrees sometimes."

"Question: Did you start with Full GAPS or Intro first? How long have you been on each?
Answer: I definitely started with Full GAPS. I knew I would be starving without starches. I ate a lot of coconut flour muffins! About a month later (November, 2010), I started intro."

"Question: What kind of progress or healing have you seen?
Answer: My mental symptoms are at least 90% better. I smile and laugh. I go on vacation. We change things around the house sometimes. I clean and put things away. I can drive and get on the freeway. Things that most people take for granted are a huge blessing to me! I'm so grateful!"

"Question: What other strategies have you tried other than GAPS? Why?
Answer: I did the "Leptin Reset," from a guy named Jack Kruse. You eat a fat breakfast and huge protein, then space out your mealtimes, and stop eating before 7:30 at night. It works on your hypothalamus to correct "upside down" cortisol levels. It helped a lot."

"Question: Are you off the GAPs diet?
Answer: No. I really like eating like this."

"Question: Are there areas where you have not seen healing so far?

Answer: I still have some anxiety, and I still have a hard time with change. But I definitely have improved."

"Question: What has been the hardest thing about following the GAPS diet?
Answer: Having to cook absolutely everything that I put in my mouth. That was really hard to adjust to. Traveling, restaurants and family gatherings are also tricky. But after almost 3 years I've gotten used to it."

"Question: What has been the best thing about following the GAPS diet?
Answer: I love the food. I'm not addicted to food anymore, but I enjoy it. But of course, the best thing is that I have a life now! I'm thankful that I get to be a better wife and mom."

"Question: Do you have any advice for a person considering going on the GAPS diet?
Answer: Join GAPS groups on Facebook and read blogs. Maybe consult a Certified GAPS practitioner if you need help with digestion."

It seems that for Debbie the GAPS Diet cleared up most of the symptoms she was dealing with: depression, bipolar disorder, and it lessened the anxiety she was experiencing without treating it in its entirety. While different people try out the GAPS Diet for different reasons, many who try it out say they see positive effects for all of the restriction and elimination involved. Weight loss is not the direct intent of the diet, but you will most likely lose weight by following the protocol just by cutting out sugar in most forms, carbs, and processed foods. When you give your body soothing and nutrient-dense foods, it will look better and run better long-term with adequate nourishment to add to an overall healthy functioning body. The correct balance of gut microbiota will stabilize your system and ensure you that you are less likely to get ill and that if you are already dealing with system issues, you will experience a thorough healing.

Chapter 2: Benefits of the GAPS Diet

Though disputed, Dr. Campbell-McBride's protocol could potentially address the following issues or have the following benefits:

1. Autoimmune Disease

Did you know that all types of autoimmunity begin in the gut? According to mindbodygreen.com, "the gut is also known as our second brain, comprised of numerous microbiota regulating and protecting the mucosal lining. When there is an imbalance, also known as dysbiosis, studies show this increases inflammation in the body and predisposes the body to autoimmune conditions." Most autoimmune diseases involve a permeable intestinal lining aka leaky gut. An inflammatory response and an antibody response are triggered by your body to attack the body's own healthy tissue and your body becomes inflamed. The GAPS Diet removes foods that contribute to leaky gut while providing the body with building blocks needed for healthy tissue.

2. Stronger Immune System

People have 4-6 pounds of bacteria in their gut, and that's also where the immune system resides. Gut bacteria that is out of balance can cause health issues like autoimmune diseases, so trying out the GAPS Diet could give your immune system a great boost!

3. Chronic Candida Overgrowth

According to the Center for Disease Control, candidiasis is an infection caused by fungal yeasts that are part of the Candida genus. "Candida yeasts normally reside in the intestinal tract and can be found on mucous membranes and skin without causing infection; however, overgrowth of these organisms can cause symptoms to develop."

While the GAPS Diet contains the natural sugars from fruit, these sugars and nutrients are an important part of nourishing the body. On the diet, you can eat natural sugars and eliminate candida infection.

4. Arthritis

In the last chapter we talked about gut flora imbalance, and that along with a leaky gut can lead to arthritis. Collagen molecules in the joints get attached to toxins leaking into the bloodstream which causes your body to launch an immune response and attack your joints. Inflammation from this immune system attack can be calmed through the use of the GAPS Diet by cleansing the body of toxins.

5. Autism

A complex condition thought to result from a combination of genetic and environmental factors, autism studies have found that up to 70% of those who suffer from autism also have poor digestive health, such as an increased risk for intestinal permeability. While no studies have been able to directly link the existence of intestinal permeability in children with and without autism, trying out the GAPS Diet could greatly improve your child's autism symptoms or even do away with their symptoms completely.

6. Depression and Other Mental Illnesses

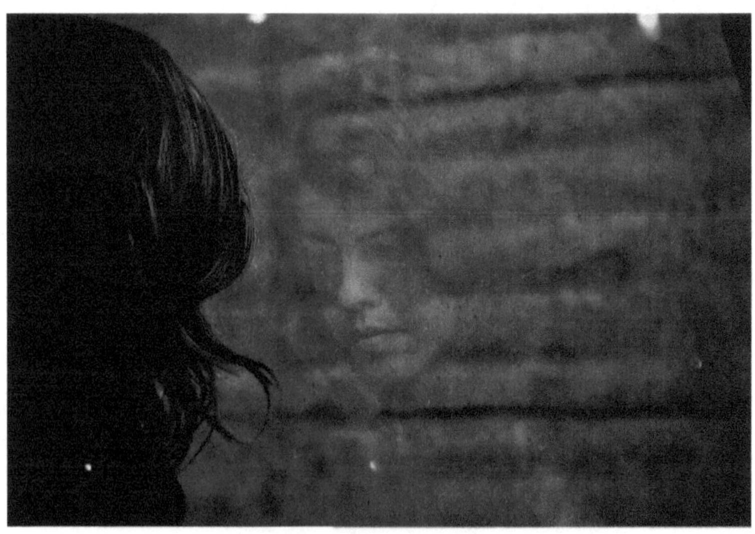

Photo by Tiago Bandeira on Unsplash

Parts of mood regulation are controlled in the gut; if we are not eating foods that are easily digestible, our body is not able to use the nutrients it needs to regulate our moods. When we are able to correct our digestion, we will be able to provide our body with the nutrients needed to function properly. Depression, OCD, anxiety, bipolar disorder, and schizophrenia may all be illness that are treatable with the GAPS Diet. The diet can affect the following aspects of mental illness:

- Neurotransmitter deficiencies resulting from impaired protein digestion and imbalanced gut flora
- Hormone imbalances tied to chronic diseases
- High toxin levels

7. Hay Fever and Allergies

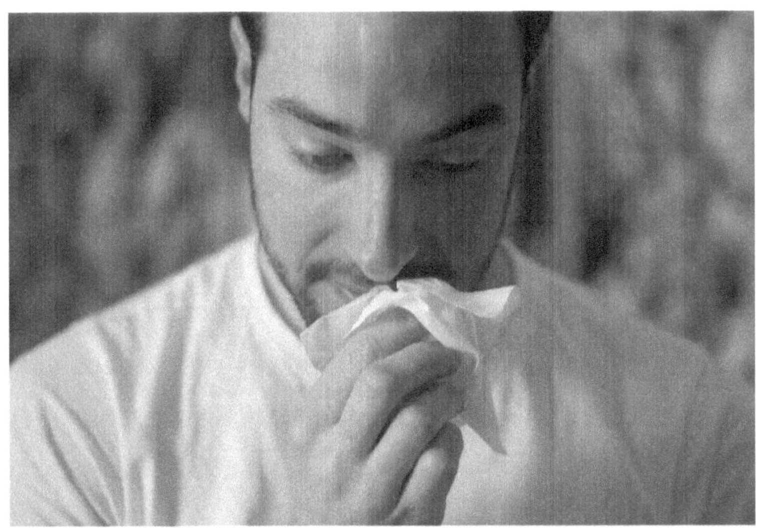

Photo by Brittany Colette on Unsplash

Histamines are produced in the body as part of your body's immune response to foreign pathogens. The gut flora plays a role in regulating this organic nitrogenous compound, so making sure your gut bacteria are in balance could have a positive effect on the allergies you experience. The GAPS Diet forces healthy bacteria production, therefore, lowering or eliminating toxins and infection from the bloodstream. When the diet is started, detoxification begins to reverse the overproduction of histamine in the body.

8. Anemia

A leaky gut lining contributes to poor absorption of the essential vitamins and minerals that support healthy iron levels, particularly in women. The GAPS Diet is able to address anemia through the elimination of contributing factors and foods that cause inflammation and add in good gut flora and supplemental nutrients that can seal the intestinal wall.

9. Eczema

While the ailment manifests on the skin, eczema is not really a skin condition, but a condition of the inner ecosystem imbalance. When there are not enough good bacteria in the gut, pathogenic bacteria are allowed to overgrow, causing leaky gut; Essentially eczema is an autoimmune condition where the skin becomes the body's target. Progressivehealth.com says "the immune system reacts to the presence of... foreign substances by releasing proinflammatory cytokines. Therefore, leaky gut can cause eczema by allowing harmful substances to reach the skin and by increasing inflammation in the deep layers of the skin."

10. Sugar Addiction

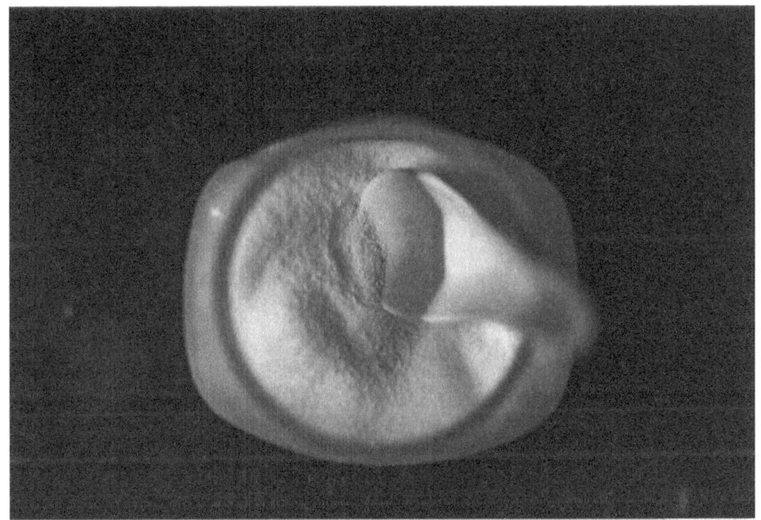

Photo by Dewang Gupta on Unsplash

The GAPS Diet aims to decrease your overall consumption of sugar from the level you are at now, down to zero. By eliminating processed sugars and preservatives, you will most likely see behavioral, cognitive, physiological, and metabolic disorders you suffer from subside or go away completely.

11. Weight Loss

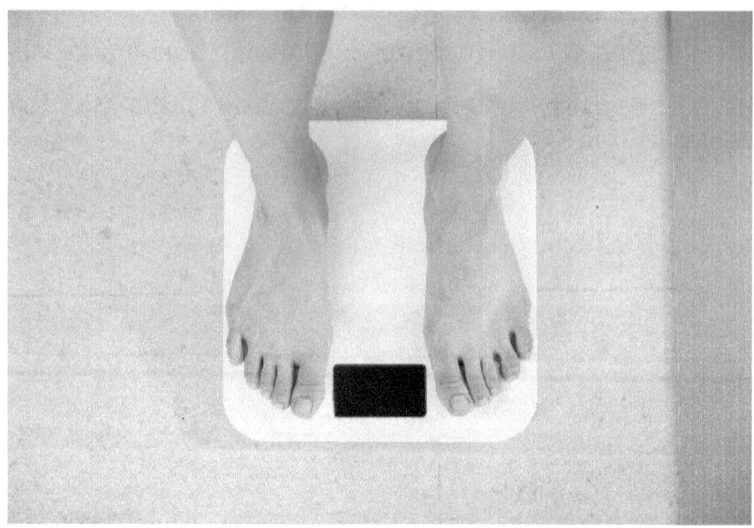

Photo by i yunmai on Unsplash

Digestive wellness plays into weight loss and weight management through gut health; Our guts house everything from bacteria (good and bad) and enzymes that help break our food down, maintain hormone production, and our immune systems that fight off infections. The GAPS Diet promotes healthy gut microbes that can reduce inflammation, insulin resistance, unhealthy fats, and more.

12. Constipation

Juicing, which is encouraged on the GAPS Diet, will stimulate bile production in the gut, which sometimes causes constipation if there is a lack of bile.

13. Celiac Disease

Celiac disease is considered an autoimmune disorder relating to gluten intolerance. Symptoms boil down to dysfunction within the digestive tract where the body has an inflammatory response to gluten that begins to damage the tissues inside the small intestine. Your body's exposure to gluten proteins can increase gut permeability leading to leaky gut syndrome. When you remove gluten and other digestive system irritants while on the GAPS Diet, you will allow your body to heal from irritation and inflammation.

Non-health related benefits can be gained from following the GAPS Diet as well, starting with a much simpler grocery list to manage on your shopping trips. Many of your foods can even be bought from local farmers markets. Make sure you always have bone broth on hand for drinking, to use when cooking, or to make soups. Your pantry will not have as many canned goods as it once did, and this diet does not require you to store anything in special containers. There will also be less baking involved in your diet unless you want to, and in that case, there are many recipes out there for GAPS-approved treats.

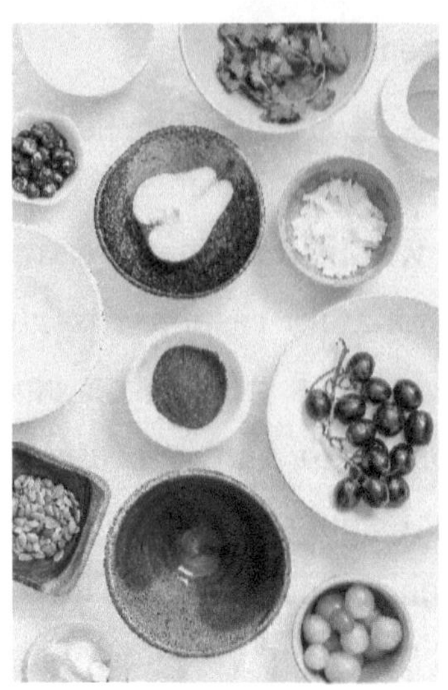

Photo by Joanie Simon on Unsplash

While you may experience life-changing benefits while on the diet, it is also easy to fall off the wagon during your journey; here are 5 ways people sabotage themselves on the GAPS Diet and how you can avoid the following pitfalls:

1. Cutting out grains but not cutting out starches
Some people will eliminate grains from their diet, but continue to each starch in the form of potatoes, sweet potatoes, potato flour, etc. While these grain-free flours are allowed, starches are a complex food molecule that are difficult for the gut to break down. Undigested starches in the stomach can begin to feed the bad gut flora, so for long-term, lasting GAPS Diet effects avoid starch along with grains!

2. Not taking a probiotic

Probiotics are important during the GAPS Diet to help reseed the gut with dominant, healthy gut flora while you starve the gut of bad flora. Finding a probiotic that is not expensive and that does the job can be challenging; to ensure you get the most out of your purchase do you research on the market to ensure your selected brand is reputable and that the brand can deliver the claimed bacterial strength.

3. Going crazy for no-grain flours

We eat a lot of grain-based foods, so deciding to cut out grains altogether can leave you confused about what you're going to be eating while on the diet. Many people will mistakenly switch from grain-based foods to the exact same foods made out of coconut or almond flour instead. For example, coconut flour is high in fiber, and if you consume too much, you may cause yourself more gastric distress, while almond flour is high in omega-6 fatty acids, but too much of this type of flour can lead to inflammation.

4. Not consuming enough broth

Consuming copious amounts of bone broth is required on the diet, preferably at every meal. All the vitamins, minerals, and amino acids reaped from the broth can soothe the intestinal tract and aid in the digestion process due to the natural gelatin content that attracts digestive juices. Make your own broth while on the diet because commercial bone broth is often watered down or packaged in toxin containers. Before you start the diet, we recommend filling up your fridge and freezer with many forms of broth you make yourself using chicken, turkey, beef, lamb, or fish bones.

5. Quitting too soon

Seeing results on the diet may take time depending on your body and its needs. For some people, it may take years for the gut to heal and return to a healthy condition, while for others it may just take months. Initial subsiding of symptoms within a few weeks or months on the diet does not mean that you are healed- you must stick with the diet to heal the gut wall and seal it for good.

CHAPTER 3: APPROVED FOODS

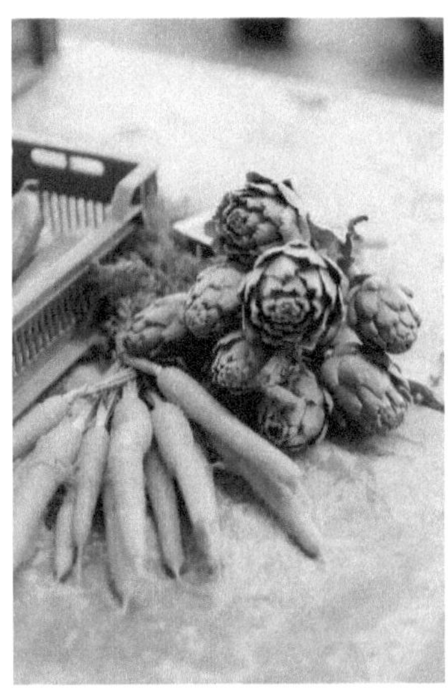

Photo by David Vázquez on Unsplash

This diet is surrounded by the incorporation of nutrient-dense, non-processed foods that have probiotic potential. While an important element is the elimination of grains, starchy vegetables, and processed carbs, the following are foods that you can eat while following the GAPS Diet:

<u>Oils, spices, etc.</u>

Almond butter or oil

Apple cider vinegar

Avocado oil

Balsamic vinegar

Basil

Brazil nut butter

Cinnamon

Citric acid

Coconut milk (homemade)

Coconut oil

Coffee

Coriander

Cumin

Butter

Fennel

Flaxseed oil

Garlic

Ghee

Hazelnuts, sprouted or as butter

Hempseed oil

Herbs, with no additives

Honey, non-processed

Macadamia nuts, soaked or as butter

Mint

Mustard

Nutmeg

Nuts

Olive oil

Peanut butter, no additives

Pecan

Peppermint

Peppers

Pine nuts, soaked or as butter

Rosemary

Sage

Sesame oil

Tarragon

Tea

Dill, fresh or drie

Cucumber

Eggplant

Ginger

Green beans

Lettuce, all kinds

Mushrooms

Onions

Parsnips

Peas

Peppers

Pickles

Radishes

Rhubarb

Spinach

Squash

Turnips

Cucumber

Fruits

Apples

Apricots

Avocados

Bananas

Berries, all kinds

Cantaloupe

Thyme

Turmeric

Vinegar

Walnuts

Vegetables

Anchovies

Arugula

Asparagus

Beetroot

Bok choy

Broccoli

Brussel sprouts

Cabbage

Carrots

Cauliflower

Celery

Cilantro

Collard greens

Raisins

Satsumas

Tangerines

Tomatoes

Watercress

Watermelon

Cherimoya

Cherries

Coconut

Dates

Grapefruit

Grapes

Kiwi

Kumquats

Lemons

Mango

Nectarines

Olives

Oranges

Peaches

Pears

Pineapple

Plums

Pomegranates

Prunes

Lamb

Lentils

Lima beans, soaked

Mackerel

Mahi Mahi

Meats- beef, pork, etc.

Pheasant

<u>Protein</u>

Bass

Beans

Bison

Cheese

Chicken

Cod

Eggs

Fish- fresh or frozen

Grouper

Haddock

Halibut

Herring

Kefir

Poultry- duck, goose, etc.

Quail

Red snapper

Salmon

Sardines

Seaweed

Shellfish

Trout

Tuna

Turkey

Venison

Walleye

Yogurt

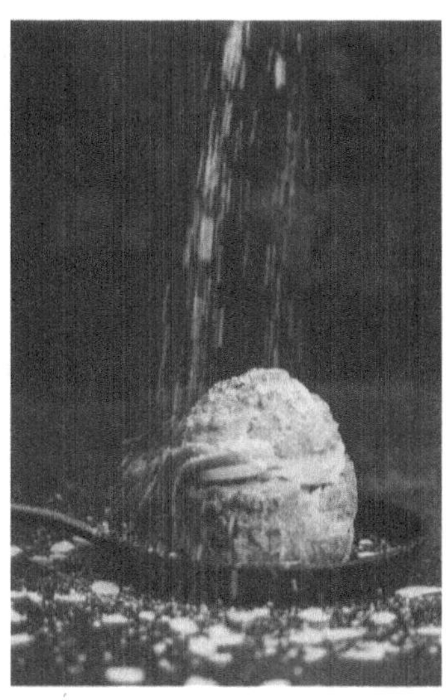

Photo by Jordane Mathieu on Unsplash

Foods to Avoid

Proteins	Black beans
Baked beans	Bologna
Butter beans	Ice-cream
Cannellini beans	Jams or jellies
Cheese- processed	Ketchup
Chestnuts	Lactose
Chickpeas	Maple syrup
Coconut milk, canned or with additives	Margarine or butter replacements
Cottage cheese	Molasses
Couscous	Pasta
Fava beans	Saccharin
Feta cheese	Soda or soft drinks

Fish- salted, breaded, or canned

Garbanzo beans

Ham

Hot dogs

Meats- processed or salted

Milk- buttermilk or rice

Mung beans

Nuts- salted or roasted

Sausage- processed

Seaweed

Yogurt- commercial

Condiments, additives, etc.

Agave

Algae

Aloe Vera

Aspartame

Baker's yeast

Baking powder

Baking soda

Bee pollen

Beer

Bouillon cubes

Brandy

Canola oil

Cellulose gum

Chewing gum

Sour cream

Sugar or sucrose

Tapioca

Tea

Grains

Amaranth

Arrowroot

Barley

Bitter gourd

Buckwheat

Bulgur

Burdock root

Cereals

Chicory root

Corn

Flour

Millet

Okra

Oats

Potatoes

Quinoa

Rice

Rye

Sago

Semolina

Soy

Chocolate	Starch
Cocoa powder	Sweet potatoes
Coffee- instant	Triticale
Cornstarch	Vegetables- canned
Dextrose	Wheat
Yams	Wheat germ

Other things to avoid include aspartame, any alcoholic beverages except the very occasional glass of wine, anything with lactose, maltose, preservatives, flavorings, colors, yeast, coffee, and soy. There are mainly three types of foods you should avoid on the GAPS Diet:

1. Carbohydrates
    a. Simple Sugars
    b. Disaccharides
    c. Starches
2. Certain dairy products
3. Processed foods

During the last stage of digestion, sugars are broken down by other enzymes, but if the gut is not functioning at its best, sometimes the necessary enzymes are not properly produced, and the sugars can't separate wreaking havoc on our system. Dairy has the same issues with sugars and the fact that dairy also contains casein. Anything else you already have a negative reaction to should be avoided while on the GAPS Diet.

You can complete this diet while adhering to vegetarianism, but you may want to switch back to meats before starting the diet. Plant foods are harder for our system to digest and can be lower in nutritional value than meats, but ways have been developed to extract more nutrition from plants and make them more digestible through fermentation, sprouting, malting, and other special ways of cooking.

There was also a study conducted in 2013 and published in the Medical Hypotheses touting the possibility that bone broth could be contaminated with lead. Bones isolate lead, which means in the process of making broth where the bones are cooked for hours may put you at risk for lead contamination; however, with this study researchers fell short in several areas leading the results to be questionable. Others may be worried about a number of other potential negative effects like an increased colonic pH levels, an increased sensitivity to foods containing artificial ingredients, and a lower number of healthy gut bacteria.

Chapter 4: How to Follow the GAPS Diet

As mentioned in Chapter 1, Dr. Campbell-McBride suggests that those who want to follow the GAPS Diet begin with the introduction phase before moving into the full diet. Starting with this part of the diet is essential if you suffer from digestive symptoms that interrupt your day like pains in the abdomen, constipation, excessive bloating, etc. This first step will quickly eliminate these symptoms and start the process of healing the digestive system. Depending on how bad of a condition you are in, you can choose to progress through the Introduction Phase in just a few days and then spend a larger amount of time doing the Full GAPS Diet.

Implementing the Introduction Phase

Each morning your day begins by drinking a small cup of water (mineral or filtered) and taking a probiotic. You are only allowed to eat the foods listed in the previous chapter; it is imperative that you do not eat anything not allowed in this phase of the diet. Taking some form of probiotic is recommended to be taken with your water.

If you think you may have an allergy to a certain food, try a Sensitivity Test before introducing it to your diet. To conduct a Sensitivity Test, take some of the food you think you may be allergic to (mash and mix with water if food is a solid), and put it on the inside of your wrist a little bit before you go to bed, making sure you let the drop dry completely before falling asleep. When you wake up take a look at the spot- if your skin has reacted to the food, stop eating that item for a couple weeks and then try the test again. If the spot does not react, you may start to gradually introduce that food back into your diet.

Stage 1: Eat homemade meat or fish stock

Meat and Fish stock will provide you with crucial nutrients for the cells in the lining of your gut; in fact, they can also provide a soothing effect on any areas where you are experiencing inflammation. Stocks that are readily available in the grocery stores should be avoided along with granules or bouillon cubes due to the fact that the cubes are full of unhealthy ingredients for our guts and are very far from their natural state.

It's actually really easy to make your own meat stock using bones, and some meat on the bone, as well as joints. The bones are very important because they provide the healing substances necessary for your gut health. To make a stock, put the joints, bones, and meat into a large pot filled with water, add in pepper and salt, bring the water to a boil, cover it, and let it simmer on low heat for 2.5-3 hours. Fish stock could be made the same way by substituting the bones and joints for the fish fins.

After 3 hours have passed, remove the bones and the meats out and strain to ensure the removal of any small leftover bones.

Any soft tissues on the bones can be collected to later add to soups, or they can simply be eaten off the bone. Extract the bone marrow from the bone while it is still hot by banging the bone on a sturdy, hard surface such as a thick wooden chopping board. Some of the healthiest solutions for the immune system and gut lining come from the soft tissue surrounding the bones and the marrow and should be eaten with every meal. The stock can be stored inside the refrigerator for up to 7 days, or if you can't get through it that quickly, you can store the broth in your freezer as well. It is preferred that you heat the stock up on the conventional oven as opposed to the microwave if at all possible.

Adding probiotics

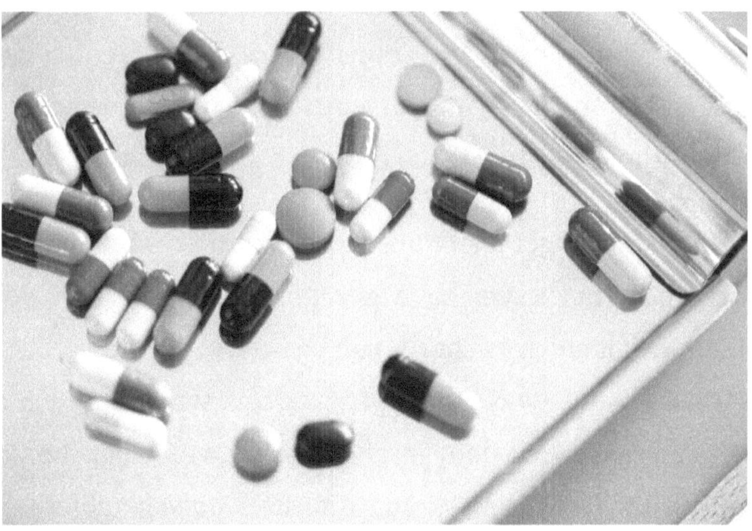

Photo by rawpixel on Unsplash

Making sure you are adding probiotics to each meal is essential right from the start of the diet. Probiotics can be dairy or vegetable-based, and you want to aim for a couple of teaspoons a day for a few days (up to 5 days) then work your way up to multiple teaspoons a day for a few days (up to 5 days) until you are able to directly take probiotics with every bowl of meat stock or soup you consume.

Stage 2: Continue with Stage 1 but add in eggs, meats, and vegetables

At this stage, you should start to add raw organic egg yolks to every container of soup and every cup of meat stock you consume. Beginning with a single egg yolk a day, slowly make your way toward eating an egg yolk with every container of broth or soup. If your body tolerates eggs well, you can start to add soft-boiled eggs to the soups. There is no need to worry about how many eggs you consume daily, in fact, eggs quickly absorb without needing much digestive assistance.

Stews can start to get introduced into your diet, but you want to ensure that the stews have a high-fat content and added probiotics. Salt and fresh herbs can be used in the stews, but you will want to stay away from spices at this stage. You will also want to increase your daily intake of homemade yogurt or kefir as well as juice from sauerkraut or fermented vegetables.

Both the Introduction Phase and the Full GAPS Diet require a very high intake of cooked saturated fats like pork, beef, etc. The broths will give you many nutrients that you would get from eating the meat, but the broth is easier on your body digestion-wise.

Stage 3: Continue with Stage 2 but add in avocado, pancakes, and sauerkraut

While continuing to eat the foods from Stage 1 and 1, you may now start to add in avocados by mashing them into your soup, starting from a couple of teaspoons and gradually increase to an entire avocado. Pancakes made from the following recipe can be consumed starting with a single pancake a day and gradually increasing:

- Organic nut butter like almond or peanut butter
- Eggs
- Fresh winter squash or marrow
- Fry the pancakes using ghee, or goose or duck fat

Eggs can continue to be consumed, and we encourage you to each not just the juices from the sauerkraut and fermented veggies but the items themselves.

Stage 4: Continue with Stage 3 but add in meats, olive oil, and fresh juices

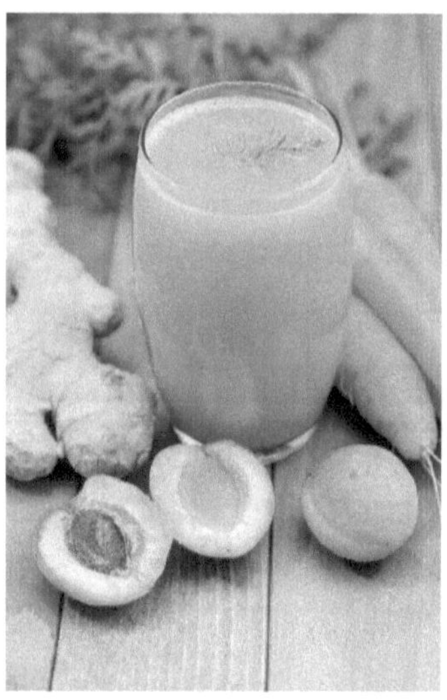

Photo by Alexander Mils on Unsplash

Gradually being to increase your consumption of cooked meats, but not yet meats that are barbecued or fried (only roasted or grilled at this point) along with cold pressed olive oil. Freshly squeezed juices may now also be added. You can start by trying a tiny bit of carrot juice; you'll want the juice you are drinking to be clear and well filtered. If the juice is tolerated well, you may drink up to a full cup a day. If you can tolerate the carrot juice, you may then start to add juice from celery, fresh mints, and lettuce, into your diet.

Juicing helps the body detox from heavy metals and other poisons collected in our body. Drinking pineapple, carrot, and a little bit of beet juice in the mornings will prepare your digestive system for upcoming meals, and it will cleanse the liver. If you do not like the taste of carrot or beet juice, you can disguise the taste by using up to 50% of the juice from oranges, grapefruits, apples, grapes, mangos, etc. The freshly extracted juices will help balance your gut's natural sugars with enzymes to produce energy for the body.

Bread you bake yourself using the following ingredients are also allowed at this stage:

- Flour made from nuts, such as almond flour
- Eggs
- Squash or marrow
- Natural fat like ghee or duck fat

Stage 5: Continue with Stage 4 and add in raw vegetables and other fruits

If everything you have eaten up to this point has been well tolerated by your system, you can add in cooked apple in the form of an apple puree. This can be cooked by peeling and coring a ripe apple and then stewing it in some water until the apple becomes soft. You can add some fat to it and push it down using a potato masher, or a fork, or you can add duck or goose fat, starting with a small amount and working your way up to more.

Raw vegetables starting with softer vegetables such as peeled cucumber or parts of lettuce can start to be incorporated back into your diet. If these are well tolerated, you may then start to add in other raw vegetables as well carrot, celery, tomato, onion, cabbage, etc. While juicing, you may start to add in apple and mango, but avoid citrus fruits at this stage of the diet. We recommend pineapple as a great juice to begin adding back in.

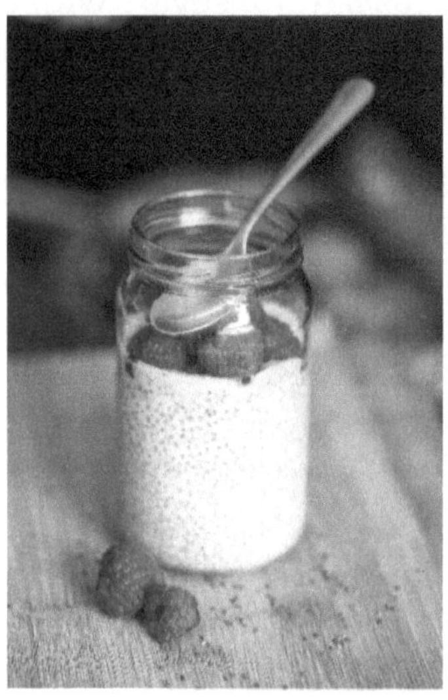

Photo by Milada Vigerova on Unsplash

Stage 6: Continue with Stage 5 and add in more raw fruit and other sweets

If everything you have tried up to this point are well tolerated by your digestive system, then you may introduce other raw fruits and some honey. Slowly reintroduce cakes made out of nut flours and other sweet things back into your diet as they are allowed at this point.

Implementing the Full GAPS Diet

If you started with the Introduction Phase, you have successfully healed your digestive system in a gentle way. If you did not start the diet in the Introduction Phase, you probably do not suffer from severe digestive symptoms, and you are able to jump right into the Full GAPS Diet.

When you wake up, start by drinking a glass of water with lemon, or press fresh juice from vegetables or fruits and dilute it with water. For breakfast, you can eat any of the following options:

- Eggs
- Sausage
- Raw or cooked vegetables
- Avocado
- Olive oil, cold-pressed
- Nuts or seeds, soaked or sprouted
- Nut flour baked goods
- Warm meat stock to drink at meals
- Weakened herbal teas with water with lemon added

For lunch and dinner, choose from the following options:

- Stew or vegetable soup
- Protein like poultry or shellfish
- Vegetables

- Avocado
- Olive oil
- Warm meat stock to drink at meals

During this phase of the diet continue to completely avoid starches and sugars including potatoes, yams, etc. and anything made out of those ingredients. Vegetables are a staple of the GAPS Diet, and they are important to eat in both cooked and raw forms; in raw form, vegetables will provide you with enzymes valuable to the digestive system and other detoxifying substances which will assist in the digestion of the meats you are eating. Raw fruits should be eaten on their own, not while you are consuming a meal because the way they are digested can make the stomach work harder than it needs to. Aim for 85% of your daily foods to be savory like meat, fish, eggs, vegetables, and natural fats. Natural fats aid in the regulation of blood sugar levels and can help you control your cravings for carbohydrates.

Pay attention to your body's pH during the GAPS Diet. Foods that are high in protein like meats, eggs, and cheese leave the body more acidic, so pairing your proteins with vegetables is essential. Vegetables are alkalizing, so they are able to cancel out the acidic effects of the proteins. Another thing to avoid is processed foods- anything packaged or found in a can. These foods a stripped of their nutrients, and they cause our digestive system to work overtime, and they can damage the balance and presence of our healthy gut flora. On top of that, processed foods are made with artificial chemicals like preservatives and colors that can be detrimental to your health.

How to Phase Out of the GAPS Diet

Begin by slowly introducing a starch you have missed during the diet, like cooked potatoes. Eating too much starch too fast may make you sick and can cause gas or stomach pain. Continue to take probiotics and drink a mug of bone broth with every non-soup meal you eat to continue to provide the gut with the building block necessary for your stomach lining. Ultimately, only introduce a food back into your diet if your body tells you it is something it wants. Change your new normal to soups, stews, animal fats, organic produce, etc. and continue to avoid sugars and processed goods.

You may add grains back into your diet, and we suggest you start with something that is gluten-free like sourdough bread. If your gut flora has been out of balance, we will have a new focus of avoiding lots of sugar in our daily diet.

Sugar on the GAPS Diet

This diet eliminates all carbohydrates unless they are carbs made of simple sugars, also called monosaccharides. The three simple sugars allowed are glucose, fructose, and galactose as they can easily penetrate the gut lining and do not need to be digested. All the fruit allowed on the diet contains sugars as well, but they should be eaten alone on an empty stomach. It should be noted that this diet attempts to pair together foods that when eaten simultaneously create glycoproteins- a slimy outer coating found on cells that accumulate in the intestine walls. Eating glycoproteins over your lifetime can prevent nutrient assimilation through the stomach lining stopping the cells from receiving the nourishment they need to survive.

Chapter 5: Recipes

Protein

Paleo Teriyaki Salmon

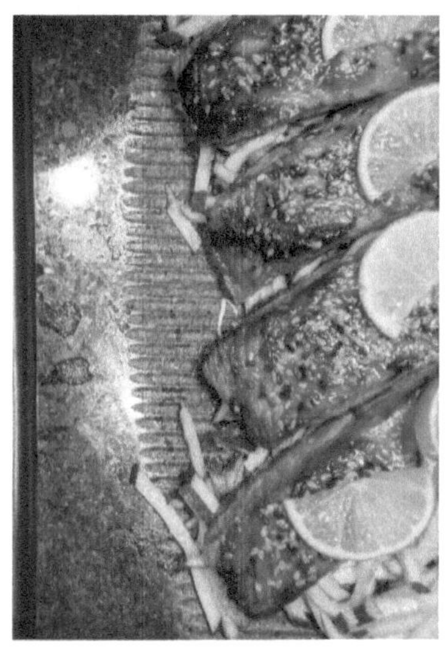

Photo by Alice Pasqual on Unsplash

Ingredients:

For sauce:

1/3 cup of tamari sauce, preferably gluten-free

1.5 tsp of arrowroot flour

¼ cup of raw honey

2 T of vinegar, coconut

For vegetables and fish:

2 T of coconut oil

1 T of sesame seeds

2 peppers, sliced

16 oz of salmon

5 green onions, chopped

Equipment:

Saucepan

Wooden spoon

Knife

Directions:

1. Combine all of the sauce ingredients into a saucepan and cook them over a low heat, making sure to stir frequently for 4-5 minutes.
2. In the pan add in 1 T of coconut oil and melt.
3. Throw in your peppers with the coconut oil and cook them until slightly brown and crisp. Remove the peppers from the stove and toss in the other tablespoon of coconut oil.
4. Cut salmon into 4 filets.
5. Place salmon pieces into the pan, and cook both sides for 3-4 minutes, or until you are sure the salmon is thoroughly cooked through.
6. Serve the salmon on a plate with the teriyaki sauce, peppers, onions, and sesame seeds sprinkled over the top.

Chicken Parmesan with Zucchini Noodles

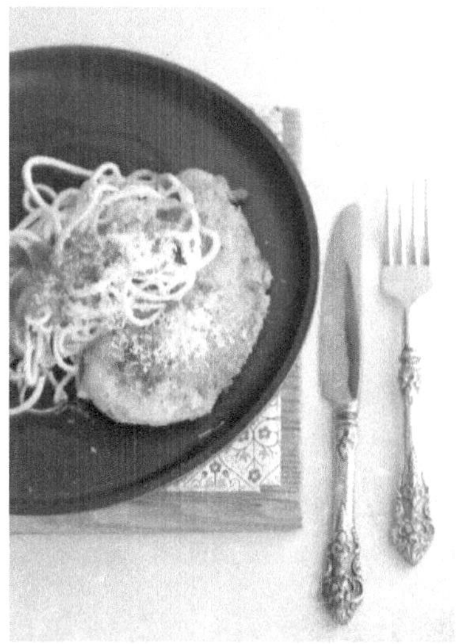

Photo from deliciouslyorganic.net

Ingredients:

For the noodles:

2 pounds of spiralized zucchini

½ tsp of sea salt

For the chicken:

4 boneless skinless chicken breasts

½ cup of Romano or mozzarella cheese

Sea salt

2 T of ghee

1 cup of almond flour

2 large eggs, beaten

For the spaghetti sauce:

1 T of extra-virgin olive oil

24 oz jar of crushed tomatoes

2 minced garlic cloves

½ tsp of sea salt

½ tsp of dried Italian seasoning

Equipment:

Colander

Paper towels

Flat-bottomed dishes

Medium bowl

Large skillet

Medium saucepan

Wooden spoon

Whisk

Directions:

1. Using a colander or a strainer, add in the spiralized noodles, toss with salt, and let the noodles sit for about 20 minutes to allow for the salt to absorb some of the water

2. Use a paper towel to blot up any excess water from the zucchini noodles and discard.

3. Preheat the broiler to high. Place flour in the bottom of the flat dish, and crack and whisk eggs in the bottom of the bowl.

4. Season the chicken with sea salt.

5. Heat the ghee using the skillet over low to medium heat for about 2 minutes, till it is melted, stirring frequently.

6. Next, we will coat the chicken in eggs first, and then flour. Dip the chicken into the eggs, and then into the flour, making sure you coat the entire piece. Place it in the skillet and repeat with all of the chicken pieces. Cook the chicken in the skillet without moving the pieces for about 4 minutes, or until the bottom of the chicken is golden brown.

7. Remove the skillet from the heat and set it on an unused burner. Sprinkle the shredded mozzarella or Romano cheese on all of the chicken pieces and broil them until the cheese has melted.

8. Once cheese has melted remove the chicken from the pan and set them on a plate.

9. Meanwhile, in a medium saucepan over middle heat, oil, and garlic. When the garlic starts sizzling, add in the tomatoes, Italian seasoning, and salt and simmer on low heat for about 10 minutes.

10. Wipe the now empty skillet down and pour in 2 T of olive oil and warm it over medium heat. Add in the zucchini noodles for 1- 2 minutes and toss them until they are hot.

11. Serve chicken with marinara and zucchini noodles.

Paleo Tuna Salad

Ingredients:

For salad:

5 oz. of tuna

1 chopped carrot

1 diced celery

1 T of brine

½ cup of coconut mayonnaise

1 chopped shallot

1 T of lemon juice

1 T of cilantro

For coconut mayonnaise:

1 egg

2 egg yolks

½ cup virgin coconut oil (melted)

1 T fresh lemon juice

1 T mustard

½ cup olive oil

¼ tsp of pepper

½ tsp of salt

Equipment:

Food processor or blender

Mixing bowl

Knife

Directions:

1. Make the mayonnaise for the salad by putting the egg and yolks, lemon juice, salt, mustard, and pepper into a food processor or blender, and briefly blend.

2. With the blender on a low speed, start slowly adding in your coconut and olive oils to the mix. Blending until all of the oil is mixed together, and there are no lumps in the mixture.

3. Combine the tuna, carrot, celery, shallot and coconut mayo in a mixing bowl.

4. Season the salad using the lemon juice, brine, and cilantro. Serve.

Hamburger Soup

Ingredients:

1 lb. of ground beef

1 cup of beef broth

4 tomatoes, peeled and chopped

2 cups of grated carrots

¼ cup of chopped onion

¼ tsp of black pepper

¼ tsp of garlic salt

Equipment:

Skillet

Knife

Wooden spoon

1. Brown the beef using a large skillet and add in the onions to begin crisping up.
2. Next, toss in the tomatoes, broth, carrots, pepper, and salt and let them all simmer together for about 15 minutes.
3. Serve hot.

Grilled Chicken with Olive Tapenade

Ingredients:

For the chicken:

4 boneless, skinless chicken breasts

Sea salt

For the tapenade:

1 cup of green olives

2 shallots, peeled

½ cup flat-leaf parsley

½ cup of extra-virgin olive oil

1 clove of garlic

1 lemon

Equipment:

Skillet

Food processor or blender

Bowl

Directions:

1. Heat the skillet on the stove top to medium, season the chicken with salt and pepper, and cook them until they are cooked through.

2. Put the green olives, shallots, garlic, parsley, lemon juice, and lemon zest in a food processor until all of the ingredients are diced. Pour the olive mixture into a small bowl, add salt to taste, and stir in the olive oil.

3. Place the chicken on a plate and top with the tapenade. Serve.

Frittata with Caramelized Onions, Sausage, and Sweet Potato

Ingredients:

For the onions:

2 yellow onions

3 T of unsalted butter

Sea salt

For the eggs and vegetables:

3 medium sweet potatoes, cubed

3 8-inch links of pasteurized sausage

12 large eggs

3 T of heavy cream

1 cup of shredded Monterrey jack cheese

2 T of ghee

½ tsp of sea salt

¼ tsp freshly ground black pepper

Equipment:

Pan

Knife

Oven-proof skillet

Whisk

Mixing bowl

Directions:

1. Preheat the oven to 400 degrees and center the rack in the middle oven shelf.
2. Cut the sausage into ¼ inch thick slices.
3. Melt the butter in a medium pan on the stove top over medium-low to low heat.
4. Season the onions with salt and cook until caramelized, for about 30 minutes, making sure that the onions don't stick to the bottom of the pan.
5. In a large oven-proof skillet, toss together the potatoes, sausage, and ghee. Place the skillet into the oven and roast for about 30 minutes, stirring occasionally.
6. Whisk together the eggs, salt, pepper, and cream in a medium bowl.
7. Take the potato mixture out of the oven, turn off the broiler, and put the skillet back on the stovetop over a medium heat. Pour the eggs over the top of the potatoes and once settled sprinkle with sausage and caramelized onions. Serve when eggs are cooked to desired state.

White Bean Chicken Chili

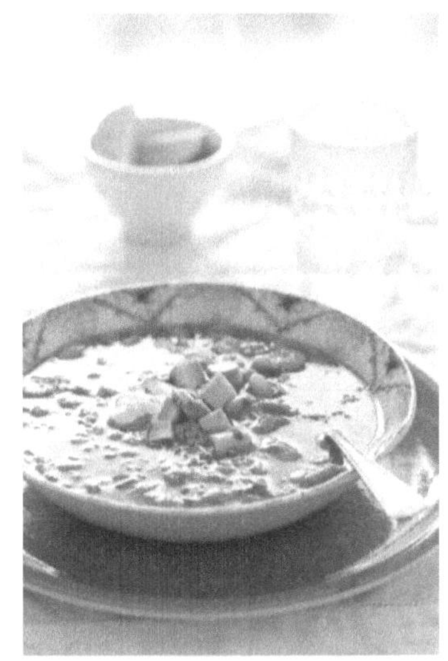

Photo from deliciouslyorganic.net

Ingredients:

4 T of unsalted butter

12 cups of homemade chicken broth

1 yellow onion

8 grilled chicken breasts, chopped

1 small pepper, preferably green

2 minced cloves of garlic

1/8 tsp of ground coriander

1/8 tsp of dry mustard

2 T ground cumin

1 T of chili powder

8 dashes of Tabasco sauce

1/8 tsp of pepper

1/8 tsp of sweet paprika

7.4 ounces of mild green chilis

2 cups of great northern beans, soaked overnight and drained

1/8 cup of tequila

16 oz jar of organic salsa

1 T of Worcestershire sauce

2 tsp sea salt

Optional toppings:

2 cups of shredded cheddar cheese

2 avocados, pitted and sliced

8 lime wedges

½ cup of sour cream

1 bunch of fresh cilantro, chopped

Equipment:

Large Pot

Knife

Wooden spoon

Directions:

1. Using a large pot over medium heat, melt the butter.
2. Core, seed, and chop bell pepper.
3. Add in the onions and pepper and cook the vegetables until they are soft (about 10 minutes).
4. Remove the pot from the heat, make a well in the center of the pot and carefully add in the garlic, cumin, chili powder, coriander, ground pepper, paprika, and

mustard. Stir them for about 1 minute until fragrant, and then stir in the tequila.

5. Put the pot back over the heat and cook for another 5 minutes or so, or until the tequila has completely evaporated. Stir all ingredients together.

6. Stir in the salsa, chilis, soaked and drained beans, chicken broth, Worcestershire sauce, Tabasco, and salt.

7. Increase the heat on the stove to high and bring the pot to a boil for several minutes.

8. Lower the heat, and let the chili simmer for 4-5 hours, or until the beans are soft.

9. Stir in the chicken breasts and serve with toppings.

Chicken Noodle Soup

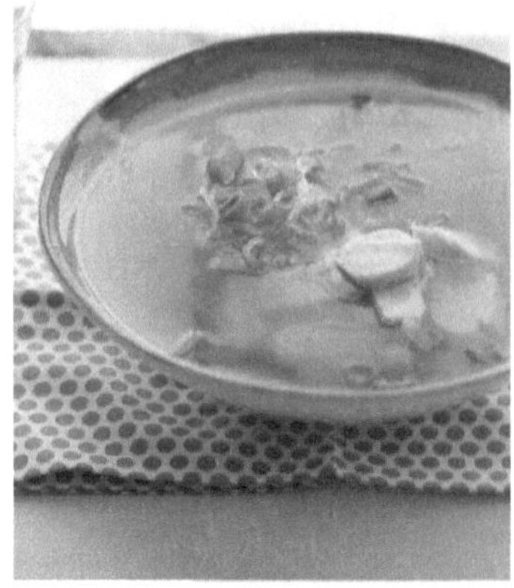

Photo from deliciouslyorganic.net

Ingredients:

2 quarts of chicken stock

6 stalks of celery, chopped

16 ounces of kelp or rice noodles

¼ cup of chopped green onion or parsley

4 boneless, skinless chicken breasts

6 carrots, chopped

Sea salt

Equipment:

Knife

Large Pot

Ladle

Directions:

1. In a large pot add in the chicken and bring the stock to a simmer. Cut up the chicken into chunks and add it along with the celery, noodles, and carrots to the pot, and cook them all for about 20 minutes, or until the chicken is cooked through. Season with salt to taste.

2. To serve, ladle into a bowl and garnish with parsley or onion.

Pizza

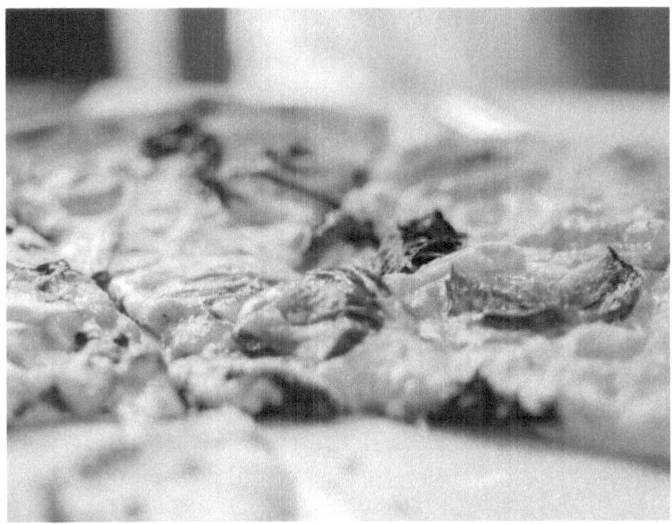

Photo by Sarah Shaffer on Unsplash

Ingredients:

For the crust:

1.5 cups of small seeds (sunflower seeds work great)

1 cup of shredded Romano cheese

2 roasted peppers, preferably red, orange, or yellow

1.2 tsp of Italian seasoning

½ tsp of salt

For the marinara:

1 T of extra-virgin olive oil

1 minced cloves of garlic

½ tsp of dried Italian seasoning

24 oz jar of crushed tomatoes

¾ cup of shredded mozzarella cheese

½ tsp of sea salt

Any other toppings of choice

Equipment:

Knife

Baking sheet

Food processor

Parchment paper

Medium saucepan

Wooden spoon

Directions:

1. Preheat the oven to 300 degrees and adjust the oven rack into the middle of the oven. Put a pizza baking sheet in the oven.

2. Using a food processor or blender, process the seeds until they are ground down to a fine powder. Add in the peppers, salt, cheese, and Italian seasoning and process until smooth.

3. Scoop out ¼ cup of dough on a sheet of parchment paper set on the counter. Spread the dough into a 6" circle and bake on the preheated baking sheet for 20-25 minutes.

4. Meanwhile, heat the oil and garlic in a saucepan over low-medium heat. When the garlic starts to sizzle, add in the tomatoes, salt, and Italian seasoning and turn the heat down to a low simmer.

5. Take the crust out from the oven, top it with marinara sauce and sprinkle with a few T of cheese and any other toppings you would like.

6. Bake for an additional 10- 15 minute, depending on desired crust crispiness and serve.

Vegetables

Carrots with Apricots, Hazelnuts, and Crème Fraiche

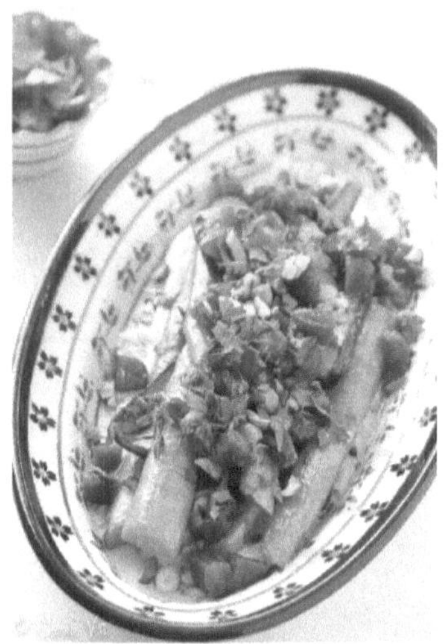

Photo from deliciouslyorganic.net

Ingredients:

For the carrots:

1 pound of carrots

2 T of unsalted butter

½ tsp of sea salt

For the apricots:

¼ cup of fresh orange juice

¼ cup of chopped and dried apricots

For the toppings:

½ cup of crème fraiche (omit if dairy intolerant)

¼ cup chopped hazelnuts

¼ cup of chopped flat-leaf parsley

1 T of raw honey

Equipment:

Knife

Large skillet

Tongs

Small saucepan

Colander

Directions:

1. In a large skillet over medium heat, melt the butter.

2. Peel and cut carrots in half length-wise and place into the skillet side by side in a later and cook them for 4-5 minutes until the edges start to turn golden brown.

3. Using tongs, flip the carrots over and continue to cook them until the other side turns golden brown. If you want your carrots to be crunchier, reduce the cooking time on each side by 1 minute.

4. While the carrots are browning, simmer the orange juice and apricots over a low heat. Take the saucepan off the heat and drain using the colander.

5. To serve, spread the crème fraiche on a serving platter, top with carrots, hazelnuts, parsley, apricots and drizzle with honey. Serve immediately.

Cream of Vegetable Soup

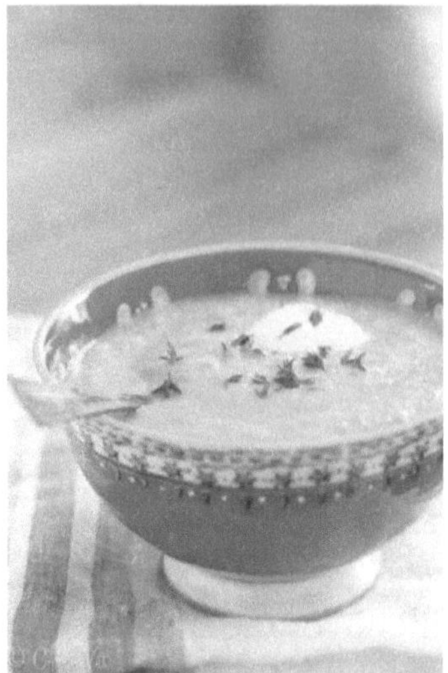

Photo from deliciouslyorganic.net

Ingredients:

4 T of butter, or 3 T duck fat for a dairy free option

2 yellow onions, chopped

4 carrots, chopped

10 cups of chicken stock

4 large russet potatoes, chopped, or 1 large head of cauliflower, chopped for a lower carb option

4 zucchinis, cut into 1-inch coins

3 sprigs of thyme, tied together with twine

½ cup of raw heavy cream

2 tsp sea salt

Crème fraiche, sour cream, or raw shredded cheddar cheese (optional)

Equipment:

Knife

Dutch oven

Hand-immersion blender or regular blender

Ladle

Directions:

1. Using a Dutch oven, melt the butter over a low-medium heat. Add in onions and carrots and put the lid over the pot to let the vegetables sweat and soften for about 30 minutes.

2. Add in the potatoes and chicken stock to the Dutch oven and increase the heat to medium-high and boil. Reduce the heat so that the potatoes and stock are at a low boil and cook the potatoes until they feel soft when poked with your fork.

3. Add the thyme sprigs and zucchini to the Dutch oven and cook for an additional 8-10 minutes- you want the zucchini to be tender. Remove the thyme bundle from the soup and discard.

4. Use a hand-immersion blender and blend the soup until it is smooth. Stir in the salt and cream. If you do not have a hand blender, you can chop up the onions, carrots, potatoes, and zucchini and blend them in a traditional blender before adding them back to the Dutch oven.

5. Ladle the soup into a bowl and serve.

Wedge Salad with Garlic Yogurt Dressing

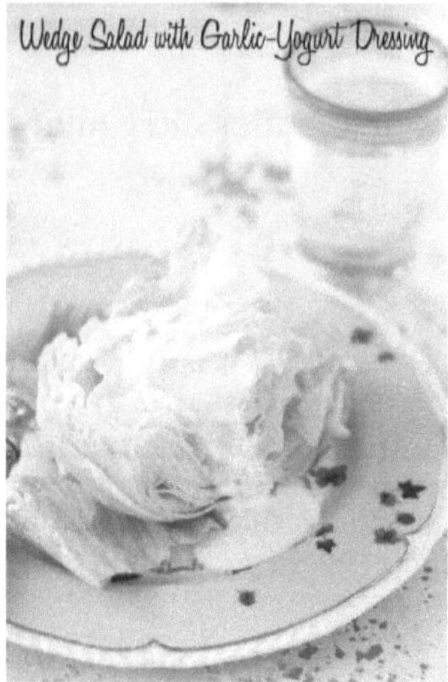

Photo from deliciouslyorganic.net

Ingredients:

1 head of iceberg lettuce, cut into wedges

1 cup of whole, plain yogurt

2-3 T of olive oil

1 clove of garlic

1 T of red wine vinegar

¾ tsp of sea salt

Equipment:

Mason jar

Hand-immersion blender or regular blender

Directions:

1. Put all ingredients into a large mason jar.

2. Using a hand-immersion blender, blend until smooth (or you can put all ingredients into a traditional blender).

3. Pour the dressing over an iceberg lettuce wedge and serve.

4. Store any excess dressing in a mason jar in the fridge.

Roasted Squash with Pumpkin Seeds, Goat Cheese, and Dates

Ingredients:

1 squash, preferably acorn

¼ cup of soaked and dehydrated pumpkin seeds

4 cloves of minced garlic

2 T of ghee or palm shortening

¼ tsp sea salt

1 cup of dates, preferably Medjool

¼ cup of goat cheese

Equipment:

Knife

Large baking sheet

Parchment paper

Tongs

Directions:

1. Preheat the oven to 400 degrees and place the rack into the middle of the oven.

2. Remove the seeds from the squash and cut them into wedges.

3. Remove the pits from the dates and cut them into quarters.

4. Line a large baking sheet with parchment paper, season the wedges with ghee and salt and place them on the baking sheet. Roast the wedges for 30 minutes.

5. Using a pair of tongs remove the squash from the oven and carefully season each piece with garlic and dates before turning each piece over and roasting them for another 12 minutes.

6. Let the squash cool for about 10 minutes. Add pumpkin seeds and goat cheese to the squash wedges as desired. Serve warm.

Green Beans with Prosciutto

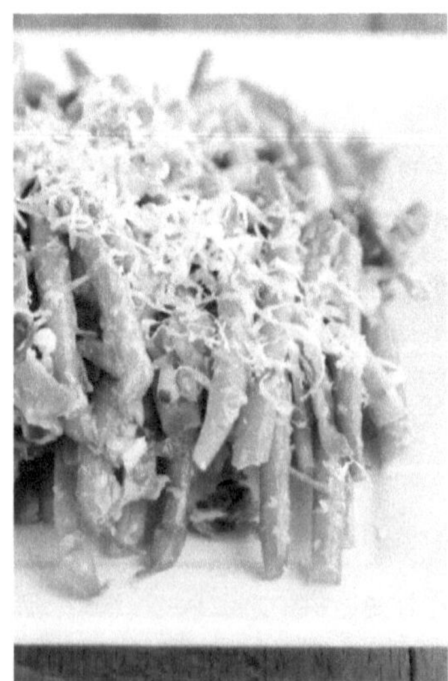

Photo from deliciouslyorganic.net

Ingredients:

    1 pound of green beans, ends trimmed

    2 T of lemon juice

    3 T of extra-virgin olive oil

    ¼ cup of minced red onion

    ¼ cup of grated Romano cheese

    4 ounces of prosciutto

    Sea salt

    Black pepper

Equipment:

    Cheese grater

    Medium pot

    Medium bowl

    Strainer

Directions:

1. Boil a medium pot of water. On the counter next to the sink fill up a large bowl with ice water.
2. Boil the beans for about 1 minute, until soft. Drain the beans, and quickly dump them into the cold water.
3. Use the now empty pot to crisp up the prosciutto over medium heat.
4. Add cheese, lemon juice, onion, olive oil, and prosciutto to the green beans.
5. Toss well, sprinkle with salt and pepper and serve.

Southwestern Stuffed Bell Peppers

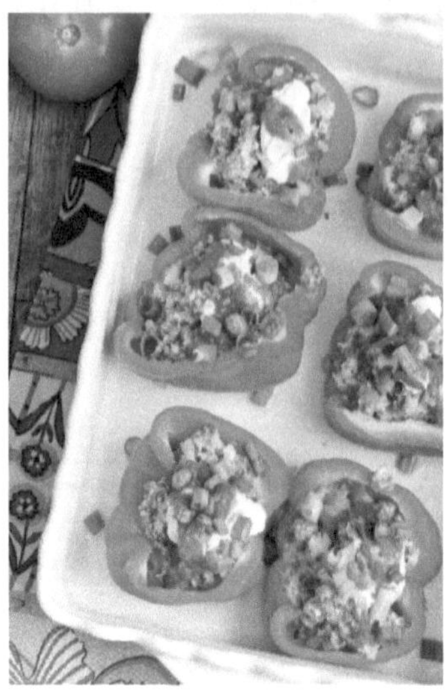

Photo from deliciouslyorganic.net

Ingredients:

2 T of coconut oil

4 large bell peppers (any color)

6 green onions

1 pound of ground beef

4 ½ oz can of green chiles

3 cups of riced cauliflower

1.5 tsp of ground cumin

½ cup of salsa

2 cloves of garlic

2 cups of shredded Monterrey Jack cheese, divided

½ tsp of sea salt

½ cup of sour cream or crème fraiche

Equipment:

> Knife
>
> Large skillet
>
> Wooden spoon
>
> Baking dish
>
> Foil

Directions:

1. Preheat oven to 375 degrees and adjust the rack to the middle of the oven. Using a large skillet over medium heat, melt the coconut oil.
2. Slice the onions and separate the white and green parts.
3. Cut the bell peppers in half lengthwise and remove the seeds.
4. Add the white parts of the onion and the beef into the skillet and cook until the beef is cooked through about 5-7 minutes.
5. Make a well in the center of the skillet and add in the cumin and garlic. Cook in the middle of the pan for about 45 seconds, then stir it in with the beef mixture.
6. Add in the riced cauliflower, 1 cup of cheese, chiles, and salt to the pan combine until all of the ingredients are incorporated. Remove pan from heat.
7. Put the peppers cut side up into the bottom of a baking dish. Divide the meat filling mixture evenly among the peppers. Add ½ cup of the water into the bottom of the pan, cover with foil, and bake for 25 minutes.

8. Remove from oven, take off the foil and put sour cream, salsa, and the remaining cup of cheese on all of the peppers.

9. Keep the baking dish uncovered and cook it for an additional 10 minutes until the cheese is melted. Serve.

Vegetable Tian

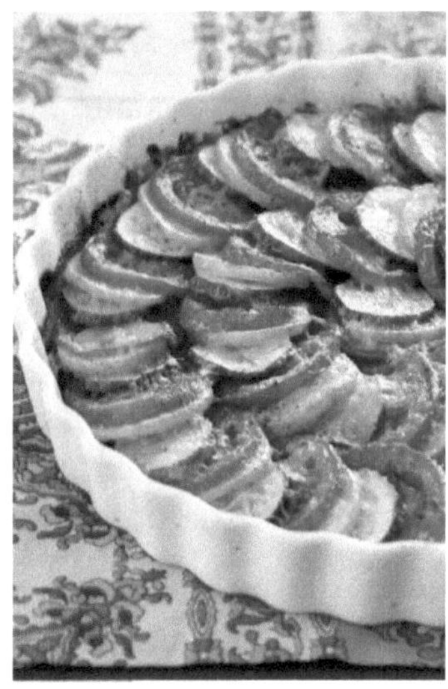

Photo from delicouslyorganic.net

Ingredients:

3 T of extra-virgin olive oil

4-5 Roma tomatoes

½ cup of grated Gouda or Romano cheese

2 large, yellow onions thinly sliced

½ tsp of sea salt

6-7 small yellow potatoes

2 minced garlic cloves

1 tsp of thyme

4 large zucchinis

Sea salt

Freshly ground black pepper

Equipment:

Knife

Large skillet

Wooden spoon

Foil

Directions:

1. Preheat the oven to 375 degrees and adjust the rack to the middle position. Using a large skillet over medium heat, add the oil.

2. After several minutes add in the onions and some salt and cook until the onions start to turn brown (about 10 minutes).

3. Cut the tomatoes, potatoes, and zucchini into thin coins.

4. Add in the garlic and thyme and cook, stirring frequently, until fragrant for about 1-2 minutes. Spread the onion mixture evenly throughout the bottom of a 10-inch baking dish.

5. Going in alternating layers, place the potatoes, zucchini, and potatoes in the baking dish. Drizzle them with olive oil and season with cheese, thyme, salt, and pepper.

6. Place a piece of foil over the dish, put it in the oven, and bake it for about half an hour.

7. Remove the foil and cook the dish for up to 25 minutes, until cheese begins to bubble. Serve.

Desserts

Coconut and Chocolate Bites

Ingredients:

For the coconut filling:

1 cup of coconut cream

2 T of organic honey

2 T of coconut oil

1 cup of coconut, shredded

1 T of vanilla essence

Sea salt

For the chocolate layer:

6 T of organic honey

½ tsp of vanilla extract

¾ cup of cocoa butter

1 vanilla seed pod

1 T of organic coffee

¾ cup of cocoa powder

Equipment:

Pan

Baking dish

Knife

Airtight container

Mixing bowl

Baking sheet

Directions:

1. Melt together all of the coconut filling ingredients in a pan over medium heat.
2. Take the coconut mixture out of the pan, put it into a baking dish, and put it into the freezer for 4-24 hours.
3. Take the mixture out of the freezer when completely cooled and cut it into squares. Store the squares in an airtight container in the freezer.
4. Melt the butter and mix it with cocoa powder in the pan over medium-low heat. Add in the honey, coffee, and vanilla and stir it continuously.
5. Take the coconut squares out of the freezer, and one by one and dip them into the chocolate mixture with a fork. Set the chocolate dipped coconut squares onto baking sheet.
6. Store them in the refrigerator for 10 minutes, or until chocolate has set and serve.

Vanilla Pudding Pops

Ingredients:

1 cup of heavy cream

¼ cup of maple syrup or raw honey

4 raw pasteurized egg yolks

2 tsp of unflavored gelatin

1 cup of whole milk (or almond for a dairy-free option)

1 T of vanilla extract

Equipment:

Saucepan

Wooden spoon

Large measuring cup

Whisk

Popsicle molds

Directions:

1. Pour ½ cup of the heavy cream into a saucepan, sprinkle in the gelatin, and let it sit for 5 minutes over medium heat.

2. Stirring constantly, dissolve the gelatin for 2-3 minutes. Pour this hot mixture into a large measuring cup.

3. Add the remaining ½ cup of heavy cream, whole milk, maple syrup, vanilla, and egg yolks into the hot cream mixture.

4. Whisk to combine the mixture and pour it between 6 Popsicle molds. Freeze.

5. Serve frozen.

Raspberry Crumble Bars

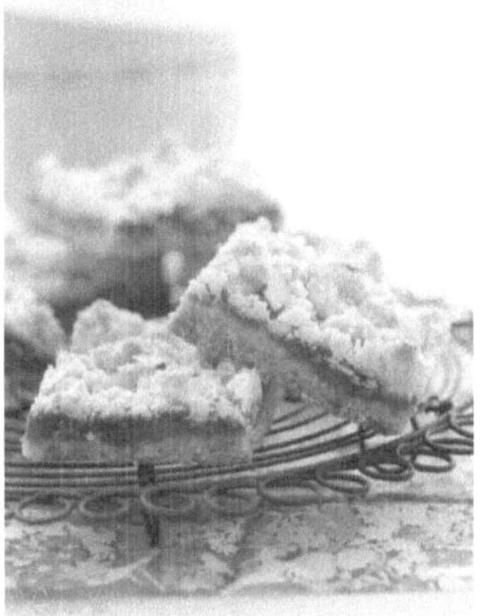

Photo from deliciouslyorganic.net

Ingredients:

For the crust:

1 T of coconut flour

¼ cup of unsalted butter, melted

1.5 cups of blanched almond flour

½ tsp of baking soda

1 T of pure honey

¼ tsp of sea salt

1 tsp of pure vanilla extract

1/3 cup of raspberry preserves

For the topping:

1/3 T of melted butter

1 tsp of pure honey

½ cup of unsweetened finely shredded coconut

¾ cup of blanched almond flour

¼ cup of sliced almonds

For the raspberry preserves:

4 cups of raspberries

1 cup of whole cranberries

1-1.25 cups of pure honey

1 lemon

Equipment:

Medium saucepan

Mixing bowls

Wooden spoon

Mason jars

8x8 inch baking dish

Parchment paper

Whisk

Knife

Directions:

For the raspberry preserve:

1. Stir the raspberries and the honey in a medium-sized saucepan while boiling over a medium to medium-high heat.

2. Keep the mixture at a constant simmer while slowly reducing the heat. Allow the berries to simmer for 20 minutes, occasionally stirring.
3. At 20 minutes, mash up the cranberries against the side and bottom of the saucepan using a wooden spoon.
4. Maintain a gentle simmer and break up any large pieces of fruit that have stuck together. After 10 minutes or when the mixture is not runny but somewhat gooey, turn the heat on the stove off. The mixture will thicken as it cools down.
5. Pour the fresh-squeezed lemon juice over the warm preserves, stir, and let the preserves cool down to almost room temperature.
6. Evenly distribute the preserves among four to six 8 oz glass jars leaving some space at the top for the preserves to expand. Freeze.

For the bars:
1. Preheat the oven the 325 degrees and put the rack in the middle of the oven.
2. Line the bottom of the 8x8 baking dish with parchment paper, ensuring that some paper hangs over the side of the baking dish.
3. In a small bowl, combine the flour, baking soda, and salt.
4. In a medium bowl, whisk together the melted butter, flour, honey, and vanilla. Stir in the blanched almond

flour mixture to the butter mixture and mix with a spoon until everything has formed a single mixture.

5. Put the dough into the baking dish as a crust. Make sure the crust is as flat and even as possible before baking. Put the crust in the oven for 5-6 minutes until you can see it start to rise and crisp up.

6. Remove them from the oven and spoon the raspberry preserves over the hot crust, spreading them evenly and leaving about ¼ inch of bare crust on all sides.

7. Use the same bowl you made the crust in to whisk together the melted butter and honey. Stir in the flour and shredded coconut until incorporated, but the dough is still a bit moist and crumbles when you touch it.

8. Crumble the coconut topping and sliced almonds across the top of the preserves. Bake the bars for 15-20 minutes, until the topping begins to look crispy. Cool the bars completely before transferring them to a refrigerator for 2-3 hours to chill.

9. Once the bars have cooled, take them out of the fridge and carefully lift the bars out of the dish and onto a cutting board. Cut into 16 square bars. Enjoy!

Pumpkin Pie Shakes

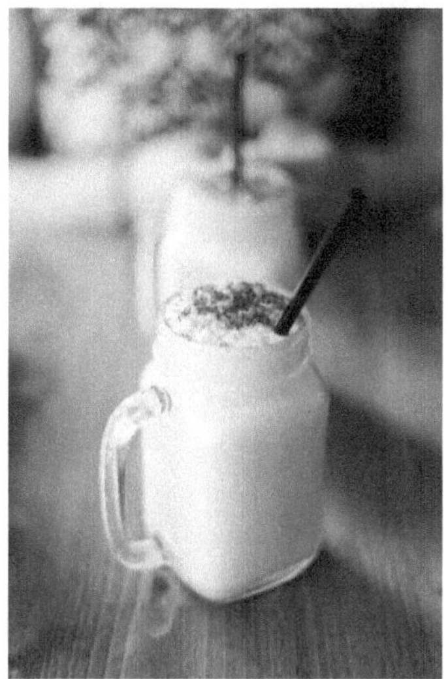

Photo by Oscar Nord on Unsplash

Ingredients:

2 cups of canned coconut milk

1/3 tsp of pumpkin pie spice

2 cups of water

½ cup of cooked and pureed pumpkin

1 tsp of vanilla extract

4 raw and organic, egg yolks (optional)

8 T of maple syrup or honey

1 cup of ice

Equipment:

Blender

Directions:

1. Place all ingredients in a blender and blend until smooth.
2. Serve immediately.

CONCLUSION

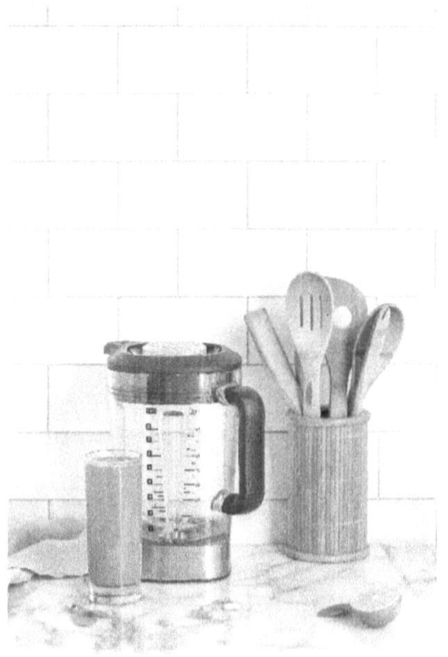

Photo by Alison Marras on Unsplash

Thank you for taking the time to read the GAPS Diet: Nutrient filled recipes aimed at Rapid Gut Repair, I know it was informative and able to provide you with all of the tools you need to achieve your goals. We hope that you now have a better understanding of what the GAPS Diet is, who the diet is for, and what the protocol is to achieve long-lasting gut health without being inundated with an abundance of old and incorrect information that takes up your time to sort through between what is fact and what is fiction.

This diet, when strictly followed, will lead you on the right path to a healthy and functioning digestive system. This diet is not low-carb or Paleo, although some recipes may fall under one of the latter categories; foods that are not allowed while on the GAPS Diet because they are hard for your system to digest.

An ideal time frame to stick to the GAPS Diet is anywhere from 1 year to the rest of your life. Some people may just choose to stay on it until their digestive symptoms are relieved, but to achieve lasting relief this diet will need to implement it as your new lifestyle; if you begin to eat grains and high-processed foods again, there is a good chance your system will return to its dysfunction. While our modern diets are high in a variety of foods that wreak havoc on our systems, we can take control of what we put in our mouths and see a different outcome from our usual sluggish and sick lives.

Integrative Nutrition quotes, "The only way to really know if this approach works is to try it out for yourself. Everybody is different. You might be thinking, isn't there a simple solution that works for everyone? The answer is no, because of bio-individuality.... each unique person has different physical, emotional, and mental needs. The GAPS Diet is no different – it may be hugely beneficial for some people, and detrimental for others. And still for others, it will be neutral – not especially helpful or harmful." Just remember that the first few days of starting anything new is the hardest! Preserve through the first week, and we guarantee your path to a healthy gut should be smooth sailing.

Finally, if you found this book useful in any way, a review wherever you purchased is always appreciated! Let us know what your experience has been like on your journey with the GAPS Diet!